HEART DISEASE & ME

A Cardiac Arrest Survival Story

RONDA L. YOUNG

Heart Disease & Me
Copyright © 2023 by Ronda L. Young

This publication contains the experiences of its author
only. It is intended for general information, and readers
are always urged to consult with their health care
providers regarding their own personal health matters.

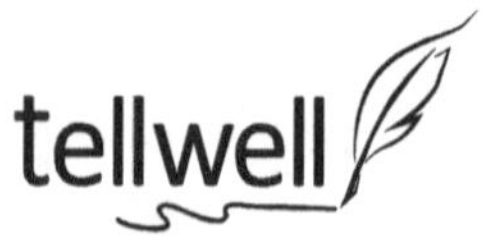

Tellwell Talent
www.tellwell.ca

ISBN
978-0-2288-8420-0 (Paperback)
978-0-2288-8421-7 (eBook)

To my sons, Jesse Hunter, and Jayme Logan, you are my purpose and my reasons 'why.' I thank God for you every single day. I love you more!

and to

My best friend, my #1 fan and greatest supporter; my loving husband, John. God knew who I needed this time around. I love you so much!

and to

My mom, dad and stepmom for all of your love and support throughout the years, I'm blessed to have you in my life.

and to

God, who has made all things possible for me, my survival, my strength, and all my blessings.

FOREWORD

I first met Ronda in 2013, when she took a First Aid course that I was teaching. Recognizing the value in what she had learned, she decided to enroll her oldest son in the Babysitting course that's offered, at a later date and location. Unbeknownst to Ronda, I would be the same Instructor teaching her son as well!

We all came together after Ronda's cardiac arrest, when Jesse was awarded the Rescuer Award from The Canadian Red Cross. I presented that award to him, and it was at that meeting, that we realized I had been both Ronda's and Jesse's instructor! Their story left me humbled and inspired!

Having First Responder training, being a Volunteer Fire Fighter and First Aid Instructor, I have witnessed first-hand the power of action and the devastation of inaction! Many freeze and are unable to dial 911, much less perform CPR. Then there is Jesse, a 14 year old boy pushing fast- pushing hard, on his mother's chest. A real life hero, who made a difference!

I will forever be grateful to have met and trained both Ronda and Jesse. Their story and the outcome of that day has continued to fuel me and my passion for First Aid training!

-Yelena Zuck-
First Responder
Canadian Red Cross
First Aid Instructor

ACKNOWLEDGEMENTS

Everyone needs a cheerleader in their lives, and I have been fortunate enough to have two. This book would not have seen the light of day without the encouragement of my wonderful husband and my aunt Joanna. Much love and many thanks to both of you, for believing in me always.

Heartfelt gratitude to the amazing cardiologists who have cared for me over the years, and continue to, you know who you are! You've given me hope and the desire to want to share my survival story. And of course Kate, thank you for being one of the best nurses a person could ever have. You've made all of my checkup appointments over the years easier with your positive outlook and caring heart.

I can't forget the reason I'm here and how this book was even possible in the first place. I owe everything to my angels. Jesse and the first responders, whom I've never met, but hope to some day. I am eternally grateful for all of you and will never forget what you did. I love you with all of my beating heart.

Your occupation is to teach others to save lives. You are the epitome of strength, determination and passion for your chosen field. Because of you, my son knew what to do on that very significant day! We are both forever grateful for you, Yelena Zuck. You make this world a better place! God bless you!

Last but not least, huge thanks to the health care team who provided me with factual medical accounts of what transpired after my cardiac arrest.

CONTENTS

Chapter One

THROUGH THE YEARS

Never in a million years did I think I would be close to death at the youthful age of 43, just two months before my 44th birthday. But this was my reality in 2014. I have heard stories of people who said they didn't think they were going to live a long life and sadly, they didn't. This was not me; I was optimistic and hopeful for a wonderful future and many more years of watching my children grow up. In fact, I would pray nightly that I would at least live long enough to see my sons get married and have children of their own. At that point in time, my boys were 14 and 8 years old; I still had so many years of watching them grow.

I had always been in decent shape. I had no health issues that I knew of, and I did not foresee any problems in that respect. I had a positive attitude despite all the things I was going through and had been through in my life.

I got married for the first time in 1998 at the age of 28, and I became a stepmom. I married someone ten years older than me and we had a long on-again, off-again relationship. Being married and having a family of my own was always something I longed for but we didn't have much in common unfortunately, and the marriage had it's share of difficulties. It remained intact for longer than it should have, but for me, it was because of the children, and the importance of family.

I remember when I was pregnant with my first child. I was scared like most expectant moms, but I was excited too, to have this little person all to myself. During this time, my marriage almost ended, yet again. This stole my joy, excitement, and anticipation, but in the end, things worked out as they usually do, and I had the most beautiful, healthy baby for whom I had prayed. Jesse was my teacher. He taught me what love is: true, unconditional love like no other. I remember I did not want anyone to touch him. I was very possessive of him because for the first time in my life I loved someone so much and I knew he loved me back. I needed him as much as he needed me. I didn't think I would ever have any more children because of my unstable marriage, but as time went on, I longed to have another little person for my son to play and grow up with. Even though Jesse had two older brothers from my husband's first marriage, the age gap was over ten years.

God blessed me again five and a half years later in

2005, when Jayme was born; another healthy, beautiful and, this time, big boy. I remember thinking crazy thoughts before he was born, wondering if I could love him as much as Jesse, but those fears were immediately erased when I saw him. My heart was full with plenty of love for both equally…I was a mom; I had a purpose. My job was to love and protect these two little beings with all I had, and that is exactly what I did. Both of my pregnancies went well with no complications. I was healthy and so were they; this was hard to believe with all the stress within the marriage. I had hoped things would improve but they never did.

I had always worked prior to getting married, I was a licensed hairdresser, but when my children were born, the thought of having someone else look after them was unimaginable to me. Fortunately, we were in a financial position where I could stay home and raise my babies. I was always thankful for that and for the lifestyle that their father provided for us.

After many years of turmoil, pain and frustration, the marriage finally ended for good in the Spring of 2013. I felt a sense of relief and freedom. I looked forward to a wonderful new beginning… little did I know this was just the beginning of more pain, struggle and being forever changed…

Chapter Two

AT DEATH'S DOOR

I was living in the matrimonial home with my two boys and two Australian Shepherd dogs, Lexy, and Chico. To say things were hard and stressful was an understatement. I was completely overwhelmed and so uncertain of the future. I knew I had to sell my home because I could not afford to keep it. I may have been free from the marriage, but I was not working, and I needed to figure things out quickly.

While the house was listed for sale, I spent months keeping it up: cleaning, mowing, shovelling and doing all the things that needed to be done. It was a lot, but I managed fine. The worst of it was all the house showings when I had to take my kids and dogs out every time until they were over.

I was able to get a part-time job and still be there for my kids for before and after school hours. I had a list of things I needed to do to prepare for a move, and one of them was to get rid of my leased vehicle. I could not afford the payments, so I had to buy something cheaper and outright. I was in ultra-downsizing mode. Despite all the pressure and decision making, I did feel happier inside than I had been, for the first time in a long time. I was hopeful still that my future would be exciting, and I looked forward to what was in store for us.

I was able to sell my home by Christmas that year, it was bittersweet. I had really hoped I could stay there but it just wasn't feasible. Thankfully, I had some family who helped me get ready to move. It was a very stressful period and I needed support without judgements, which wasn't always the case. All I needed was love, understanding and compassion with that support. It is hard to find that in people all the time but thankfully I find those things in God always. He is always there for me guiding me through the difficult times.

My closing date was January 31st, 2014. Moving in the winter sucked, for lack of a better word, but again, I managed. I had hired movers, but I made several trips myself to my new rented place to take over fragile items that I did not want damaged. I was extremely tired, which was to be expected. Being a full-time single mom with two kids and two dogs while trying to do it all, must have been taking its toll. I remember having a dizzy spell on two separate occasions while I was at work, but I didn't think anything of it. I reasoned that I was stressed and tired from all the pressure I had been under the last year and from all my responsibilities. Maybe I needed something to eat? Or drink? Or more sleep? Again, I never thought too much about it because I was healthy and in good shape.

On Valentine's Day evening, just two weeks after I moved into my new place, I volunteered to work because I was single, and I didn't have any plans. I felt fine and I went home after work and enjoyed some chocolate with my boys. I had spent the previous two weeks, hanging pictures and mirrors, trying to make our new place feel like home. I did enjoy my sweets from time to time but that was my worst habit as I did not drink, smoke, or do drugs.

The place I lived in was small, it was a two-level duplex. The primary bedroom was downstairs with another bedroom, while the third bedroom was upstairs and that's where Jesse slept. Jayme's room was still full of boxes and not set up yet, so he was sleeping in my room until it was ready. After a long day, I was looking forward to bedtime, and I went to sleep that night as per usual.

The next morning, on February 15th, I woke up early and went upstairs while Jayme was still sleeping. Jesse was playing his video game in the living room. I let the dogs out after I cleaned up the mess on the floor, that one of them had made. It was a very cold and snowy morning, I came back inside, walked up the stairs and went over to sit in the recliner chair near Jesse. I hadn't even taken my coat off. I was very tired, which is how I felt often, and the last thing I remember was resting my head in my hand and saying out loud, "I can't take much more of this…"

I woke up in the hospital the next evening. I had no memory of what happened after I spoke those words and would later be told what transpired after I did.

I had collapsed from my chair to the floor, suffering a sudden cardiac arrest (SCA). Jesse, at just 14 years old, immediately called 911 and performed cardiopulmonary resuscitation (CPR) until paramedics arrived. They arrived within five minutes and continued CPR and administered three shocks with the paddles. I was then taken to the hospital and put into an induced therapeutic hypothermia for 24 hours with intubation, sedation, and cardiac catheterization – in other words a medically-induced coma. I had gone into VT/VF which are dangerous, life-threatening arrhythmias known as ventricular tachycardia and ventricular fibrillation. After many tests with mostly normal results except for an ejection fraction (EF) of 20% the doctors were stumped as I had no cardiac arrest factors. They concluded that I, an otherwise healthy woman, had dilated non-ischemic cardiomyopathy. They said that my heart was enlarged and extremely scarred and that a virus must have attacked it at some point. There was nothing in my system at the time to indicate what that virus was.

At one point my immediate family had no idea if I was going to make it or not. Doctors as well were uncertain if I would pull through and what state I might be in, if or when I did.

Through divine intervention, Jesse's quick thinking and the quick response time from first responders, my brain function was saved. Permanent brain damage can occur after only four minutes without oxygen, and death can occur as soon as four to six minutes after that.

Approximately one out of ten people survive at-home cardiac arrests. It is nothing short of a miracle that I survived that day. When I think about the image of me lying on the floor and my son doing what he did without hesitation, it brings tears to my eyes. How he must have felt in that moment and how things could have gone that morning haunted me for some time.

When I started to wake up the next evening, I still had the breathing tube in place and they decreased my sedation. I started following commands such as squeezing hands and wiggling toes.

I tried to rip the tubes from my face and chest; I believe I was in a state of panic, I thought… *Where are my kids? I need my kids. What about my dogs?* Sedation was increased and again decreased throughout the night and turned off the next morning. I was extubated and started talking at 10:30 that morning.

When I started talking I was asking many questions but somehow knew that it was my heart. It was very strange because I had no idea anything was wrong with my heart. I knew that I had endured a lot of heartache over the years, but I had no previous diagnosis of any heart related disease. I had delivered two healthy babies with no issues, and throughout my life I lived a healthy lifestyle in which I wasn't restricted in any way.

My family suspected that I had suffered from takotsubo, which is known as 'broken-heart syndrome.' Takotsubo is stress-induced cardiomyopathy. They knew all the difficulties I had experienced over the years and wondered if that is what damaged my heart. I certainly felt that it was a possibility as stress is extremely hard on the body and can cause many illnesses. Doctors were not convinced that was the cause though.

Jesse, without a question, was my lifesaver that morning. How incredible, that I gave him life and he in turn saved mine. I would not be here today had he not acted so bravely and quickly. Ironically enough I had enrolled him in a babysitting course the year before because I wanted him to know what to do in an emergency, if he and his little brother were home alone. I did not, however, ever expect him to use that knowledge on me. At just 14 years old, he was awarded three different life-saving awards and I could not be prouder of him. I cannot stress enough how important it is to know CPR. CPR can save a life; it saved mine. I was at death's door, but it wasn't my time…

I was told that Jayme played a key role too as he let the first responders in and put Lexy and Chico away in the bedroom so they wouldn't be in the way. He also gave the police officers contact information and answered some questions. One of the officers asked my kids where my medications were. They told him that I didn't take any; they said that I didn't like taking any kinds of medications.

My mom doesn't drive and my dad was in Florida at the time, so my boys thought of their aunt right away. She was called immediately because she was a close contact and an RCMP officer. She came right away to be there for my kids, and she played a paramount role in managing my affairs until I was released from the hospital, approximately two weeks later. I am forever grateful to her for all she did for me and my boys. Something needed to be done about my dogs; they needed someone to look after them right away. My mother-in-law, at that time, with whom I was always close, offered to take them, and what a blessing that was.

Throughout it all my mother prayed faithfully, holding my cross that I always wear around my neck. She was beside herself, always a worrier when it comes to her children and grandchildren. Her prayers were a blessing, as well as others who kept me in their prayers.

Chapter Three

THANKFUL TO BE ALIVE BUT STRUGGLING TO LIVE

Several days after my SCA, while still in the hospital, I was fitted with an Implanted Cardioverter Defibrillator (ICD). I was told without it, if I had another life threatening arrhythmia and no one was around, I would certainly die. An ICD is an internal defibrillator, its job is to detect and stop irregular heartbeats. It continuously monitors one's heartbeat and will deliver shocks to restore a regular heart rhythm when necessary.

All I could think about was... *So, is this what I have to look forward to?* I became very depressed and could not be happy about my future at that point. *Why me? Why did this happen?* I had experienced low points in my life before but not like this. I had to have a psychiatric consultation while in the hospital because of my low mood, which is completely normal. The doctor reiterated how normal it is to feel depressed, educating me on the possibility of depression being the norm in the future as well. Many people can have PTSD after an event like this occurs, either a bystander or the person who actually had the cardiac arrest. I was not prescribed medication for my state of mind at that time, and I tried very hard to cope with this new reality on my own.

I had a few visitors in the hospital; friends, and some family. I struggled with my memory during that time and for some time after, so I did not remember all who came. Only immediate family were allowed to see me when I was intubated and I was told later that my two stepsons came to see me then, which touched my heart because I hadn't been in contact with them for quite some time. Also, a friend I have known since childhood visited me during recovery and it felt good to learn that these people and others were there for me.

I was educated in the hospital regarding heart health and diet, although my diet had been okay, it could always use improvement, especially now that I had a form of heart disease. I received lots of information from a dietician for me to take home. I later enrolled in a program called Cardiovascular Hearts In Motion. This twelve week program was phenomenal, it included exercise and lots of education regarding cardiovascular health.

I played in my mind over and over... *What if I had stayed in bed longer? What if it had happened the morning before, on Friday?* My boys would have been in school, and I would have been home alone; I would have been found deceased. *What if I had stayed outside longer with the dogs?* Jesse would not have realized the time. *What if he had still been in bed? What if I had been driving?* There were so many what-ifs but thank God things played out the way they did. The fact that I fell onto the floor was incredible too, because had I remained seated, Jesse may not have realized what happened.

Sudden cardiac arrest needs immediate attention. Without intervention, you will die – your heart stops beating – it can happen to anyone, at any time, at any age, without warning. I would not be here today without divine intervention; Jesse's quick thinking, the first responders, many prayers and of course the amazing health care workers at the hospital. All first responders, nurses and doctors deserve medals for what they do every day.

So, here I was a different person. I could not work, I could not drive, I had a device in my chest, and I was on several medications to keep me going. I was thankful to be alive of course, extremely thankful, but upset too. I was at the lowest I could be, I wondered why I had survived if life was going to be like this. It took some time for me to try to turn my thought process around. I tried to be grateful, but it was not easy, this was not the life I had been hoping for.

My kids were always my driving force, and I knew that I had to be strong for them. Although I was down,

I was indeed happy to still be here for Jesse, Jayme and my furkids. People would ask me constantly how I was doing; my response for several months was "I'm still here" accompanied with a shoulder shrug. In other words, I was here, but that's about it. I was not living; I was existing. I did not have the energy to do all the things I had done before. I was scared, I did not know what to expect and I felt bad for my kids that I could not be there for them like I had been in the past.

The meds made me tired and I had to learn how to live with the device in my chest. I hid it and the scar always; I did not like it or the constant reminder. It was uncomfortable. It took time to adjust to it, and I developed what is called 'frozen shoulder', which was temporary, thankfully. After the alotted time in a sling for healing purposes, and to avoid the risk of lead displacement, I barely moved my left arm, in fear of somehow still damaging the device or the wires attached to it. This is unlikely after several weeks of healing, and you should actually move your arm normally to avoid any mobility issues like I had. My ICD is placed below my left collarbone, and I could not lie comfortably on that side for several weeks. I wished over and over repeatedly that I never suffered a cardiac arrest. Now, suddenly, I had to have blood work done regularly; I had to have checkups and other tests. I was once healthy and now this. When people say that life can change in the blink of an eye, they aren't kidding. I had to rely on people to do things for me and drive me places because when you have a cardiac arrest, your right to drive is taken away for six months. If you can go six months without going unconscious from a life threatening arrhythmia, and getting a shock from your ICD, then you can automatically drive again.

Things became even more difficult than they had been before this. I still had two kids and two dogs to look after by myself and I didn't know if I could do it, but I did. I remember a couple of people suggested that I rehome my dogs even before this happened, but that was not something I could do; they meant the world to me, and they were a part of my little family. I felt that somehow, I would be able to do it all; I just had to keep having faith that things would work out. My faith is what got me through, it had always gotten me through difficult times throughout my life. The fact that I was still here meant God wasn't finished with me yet, and I prayed daily for strength and his guidance.

My new normal became being home even more than I had been before. I did not return to work because of my condition. I have always been a homebody, but this was taking it to a new level. I went on disability which was a godsend because I don't know what else I would have done at that time. My kids, a few friends and certain family members were so helpful with day-to-day chores and with anything at all that I needed. I was given food and monetary gifts, which I'm forever grateful for. A lady I didn't even know, dropped meals off for me and my boys after she heard what happened. Some people are just so kind and thoughtful and truly make this world a better place.

Despite everything that I was going through, I was indeed happy that I got to celebrate my 44th birthday in April. That was a day that almost didn't happen. Every birthday, special occasion, and milestone from now on meant more to me than it ever had. I realized through experience now, that you cannot take life for granted because tomorrow isn't promised.

We moved Jayme's bed up to Jesse's room right away and we all slept in the same room: them in the queen bed and me in the single one. We were all clearly shook up by what had happened and needed to be close to each other to feel more at ease. One day at a time became my new motto; I did not know what the future held but I knew that I had to figure out a way to live with this situation the best possible way I could. My kids were depending on me, and I could not let them down, not ever.

One thing I kept going through in my mind was *What caused this?* They said a virus. I remembered I had a few cases of strep throat over the years and was supposed to get my tonsils out, but never did. I also remembered that back in 2012 an outdoor cat had bitten me. The cat was after my puppy Lexy, I had her on her leash on our front lawn and the cat came over and started attacking her. It was the strangest thing. I picked Lexy up and it lunged at her again, but it bit me on my bare leg instead. Terrified at what just happened, I ran in the house upset and tried to clean the area as best as I could. I should have gone to the hospital but instead, I waited until the next day to see my family doctor, who prescribed an antibiotic for me. I was genuinely concerned about my health after that, and I developed a fear of cats from that point on. My cardiologists didn't seem to think either of those things could have caused what happened to my heart, but I could not stop thinking about it. What if stress, strep throat, or the cat bite had changed my life forever?

Chapter Four

SHOCKED

I had attracted some attention through the media because it was suggested that I share my story and highlight what my son Jesse had done to save my life. We were in the newspaper and on the news a couple of times; it was great to bring awareness to people about what happened. I had even started to do some volunteer work for the Heart and Stroke Foundation; mainly speaking engagements to tell my story.

Many people think that a heart attack and cardiac arrest are the same thing, but they are quite different. The easiest way for me to describe them is by comparing plumbing to electrical. A heart attack is like plumbing in the sense that your arteries can be blocked/clogged like pipes can be, which will rob the heart of its vital blood supply. Depending on the severity you may be able to still function to some degree, but immediate attention is important; as sometimes a heart attack can lead to cardiac arrest. A cardiac arrest is when your heart suddenly and unexpectantly stops beating, like a car that stops running: the battery is dead, and it will not go anywhere, hence the electrical analogy. You will not be able to function at all, and immediate intervention is necessary for survival.

I remember, at my first, of many checkups I had at the Heart Function/Transplant Clinic. I said to one of the nurses, "I can't believe I had a heart attack."

She said, "You didn't" and then went on to explain the difference to me.

I wanted to know what ejection fraction meant as well since mine was 20% at the time of my SCA. She explained that EF is a measurement expressed by the percentage of how much blood the left ventricle pumps out with each contraction. A normal EF is between 55% and 70%; a percentage of twenty or lower is indicative of severe heart failure. It is important to understand that, as mentioned before, cardiac arrest can happen to anyone, anywhere, and the survival rate is significantly lower if it happens out of hospital. I cannot stress enough the importance of automated external defibrillators (AEDs) and how they should be more prevalent everywhere — at sports facilities, shopping malls, schools, and office buildings, to name a few locations. Survival rates will increase if they are more readily available.

It was nearing Mother's Day and I was excited to spend that special day with my boys. I was trying hard each day to take my mind off of my condition and to focus on other things. On Friday, May 9th, I went to bed that night with no issues. I felt fine, and was looking forward to going to the movie theatre the next day for the first time in a long time. I woke up early on Saturday morning, I remember waking up suddenly and my boys were standing over me, asking me if I was ok. I said I was and told them that I must have been dreaming. I laid back down for a bit and then finally got up and went about my day. I went to the theatre as planned and had a great time. The next day, on Mother's Day, I had some lobster and enjoyed the day with my sons. It was a great weekend… or so I thought.

On Monday, my boys would go to school, and I would stay home and try to do what I could to make the day go by a little faster as most of my days were quite lonely, depressing, and boring. I got a phone call at approximately 8:15 a.m.; from the hospital, the device clinic to be exact. They told me I had a shock early Saturday morning for VT and that I had to come in… I cannot explain how I felt in that moment exactly, but I can tell you that it wasn't good. I had to make plans for my boys in case I was admitted that day to the hospital.

The hospital had been notified of my shock because I have a monitor in my bedroom that records data from my ICD for arrythmias and/or shocks, it is a remote monitoring system that allows the hospital to monitor a patient's condition through digital technology. The device clinic is closed on the weekends, but the staff was notified once they returned to work on Monday morning. This was my first shock and that is why I woke up suddenly on Saturday morning… I hadn't realized that was why until they told me so.

I got a drive to the hospital and was given the upsetting news… I would be admitted for testing and another six months was added to my no-driving rule. I had been slated to drive in August but now I could not drive until November. I was shattered; I had been looking so forward to driving again… It was like one step forward and two steps back.

Once I was admitted, I was scheduled for tests to be performed, tests like an EKG, echocardiogram and blood work. At this time, another medication was added to my routine which I was nervous to take. I am always nervous trying new drugs as I don't know how I'll react to them. It was an antiarrhythmic drug, which came with side effects that ended up being hard for me to deal with. I had to have frequent tests to keep an eye on my liver, kidneys and lungs from being on this medication. I was feeling defeated again. Not feeling well, being tired from the meds, being shocked and the news of a longer driving suspension, were all too much. Fortunately, the drug wasn't forever, it was only temporary to try to stop the ventricular arrhythmias I was having. My boys were understandably upset and scared and unsure of what the future held for their mom, I was very concerned about them and how they would deal with all that was happening.

I began to long for a partner to help me through these challenging times. I was still young and had a lot of years left to live…hopefully. The problem was I didn't feel worthy. My inner dialogue was telling me I was far from a catch… *I have no job, I cannot drive and I have a major health issue.* I felt like no one would want me. My lack of self confidence was worse than it had ever been. Thankfully, my depressing thoughts never got to the point where I had to be medicated. I knew I had a strong mind because I had endured so much, and I was still standing. I never turned to negative influences and always stayed in faith.

Day by day, I tried to remain positive, but I had a lot of anxiety regarding the shock. I've heard of some people describing a shock like it is a kick to the chest, but I never felt anything because I was asleep. I was so thankful that my device worked and woke me up that morning, of course, but I was scared to have another shock. The ICD was no doubt my insurance policy now and I was extremely grateful for it. I had no choice but to keep going for my kids' sake: they needed me, and I needed them just as much.

After my initial cardiac arrest and now a shock, I did not feel comfortable living where I was. I felt like I had to move; my place was a constant reminder of what had happened there. A friend of mine told me about a rental coming up a couple of doors down from her and

I jumped at the opportunity to rent it. I was lucky that the property owner told me I could have it, so I decided to move yet again for June 1st. My current landlord at the time was more than fair and understanding of my situation and allowed me to get out of the lease early. I am sure some people thought I was crazy because it was so much work to move again, but it was something that I had to do.

The move went well, and I loved it there; it was bigger and had all of our bedrooms on the same level. My biggest concern was the steep stairs. I was nervous about getting a shock from my ICD while going up or down them, it would not end well if I did. Having a friend close by eased some of my anxiety and it was so wonderful having her and her kids keep us company.

Weeks went by and I started to think about trying to put myself out there to meet someone. Hesitantly, I joined a dating site after I moved. I wanted to look around, even though I had thought that was something I would never do, but being home so much, I did not have too many options other than online dating. I was at home more than I was out, and I had been informed that Prince Charming was not going to fall through my ceiling. There were a couple of interesting people who caught my attention, so I decided to be brave and entertain the idea of meeting them. I had lots of messages to sift through to see who a good fit for me might be. I struggled with whether I should tell them about my condition or not.

I felt that being honest and up front was the best, so I did tell most of the people I spoke to. Some did not care and others said, "Good luck to you." It was not an easy process, but I hoped it would be worth it.

I arranged to meet someone at a coffee shop on July 10th. I was so nervous, but my friend who drove me said she would come in with me and sit nearby. I walked through the door of the coffee shop, with her ahead of me. I told her I felt dizzy, and the next thing I knew, I was waking up on the floor of the entrance. I had passed out and received my second shock, exactly two months after my first one. I had gone into VT/VF and thankfully my device did what it is designed to do. Thank God for my ICD! I did not feel this shock either as I went unconscious first. What made this situation even more crazy was that there was a man holding the door behind me, for the paramedics. I mouthed to my friend, while I was still on the floor, "Is that him?," meaning my date, and she said "Yes." *I was mortified.* He was still holding the door open as I was wheeled out on the stretcher and I said to him, "I'm so sorry," and he just said, "It's okay," and away I went. I didn't know whether to laugh or cry, but God love him, he messaged me later to see if I was okay and to tell me that he still owed me a coffee, which I don't drink. I am a tea drinker, and of course everything had to be decaffeinated now. I did not see or talk to him after that. I felt like what happened might be a sign, plus I was really embarrassed. I wasn't sure about trying to meet someone again after that experience, and I wondered if my anxiety about going on a first date had brought this situation on. I never did go back to that coffee shop either, even though I drive by it all the time.

So, away I go to the hospital again for more bad news, more tests, medication tweaks and no driving for another six months. At this point, I really felt like someone had put a curse on me or I was being tested, either way, I felt so defeated! I tried so hard to have a cheerful outlook and make the most of this deck of cards I was dealt, but it was not getting any better or easier. Now I could not drive until January of the next year. *Are you kidding me?*

I had a decision to make. I could wallow in self-pity, or I could try to make the most of a very tough situation. Spending time in the hospital was no fun in the summer; I wanted to be out and enjoying life. It always seemed like I was the youngest patient on the cardiac floor. A lot of patients came and went because they were in for different surgeries to fix their problem. My situation wasn't fixable, unfortunately. My coronary arteries were clear, but my heart muscle was damaged with extensive scarring, which affected its ability to function normally.

This time in the hospital, the cardiac team started to do a workup for a heart transplant. They knew that if this kept happening, I would need one. I had all kinds of tests done, one in particular was called a PET scan, this test determined that my non-ischemic cardiomyopathy was likely attributed to sarcoid cardiomyopathy. Sarcoidosis is a disease that is characterized by the growth of collections of inflammatory granulomas. It can affect many organs in the body. Cardiac sarcoid is rare and I was started on a steroid drug at this time to help with the active inflammation within my heart. I talked to many people who came in my room to discuss anything and everything about my health history. I did receive some positive news, though, that my blood type is the universal recipient. This meant that, if a transplant was needed, I could receive a heart from anyone, which is the ideal situation. I left the hospital days later feeling very scared, I remember all I could think about was possibly needing a new heart. I prayed even harder that it would not come to that; I wanted my heart to get stronger, not weaker.

I was happier in my new place and I didn't receive my shock at home, so my feelings did not change about living there. I continued on and tried the dating thing again after several weeks but realized, having no success, that it would be hard to meet my match.

As 2014 was nearing its end, I could not believe all that I had been through that year, it was surreal. Losing my home, suffering a cardiac arrest, moving twice, unable to drive or work, and receiving two shocks from my ICD… The year before was bad enough, trying to keep things together for my kids' sake but this was unbelievable…

At Christmastime, which is my favourite time of the year, we had an unexpected visit from old neighbours of ours. They brought us the most generous and thoughtful gifts; this was such a huge help, and I will never ever forget their generosity. It was such a pleasant ending to an extremely difficult year.

Finally, January 10th, 2015, came, and I COULD DRIVE AGAIN. I was SO EXCITED; I cannot explain how excited I was. ELEVEN MONTHS of not driving was incredibly hard on me. Finally, no more relying on other people for drives. I had my freedom back and I prayed that I would never need another shock from my ICD again. Initially, I was afraid to drive, of course, wondering if I would have a shock while I was driving, but I had to push through those thoughts. I did not want my anxiety to steal my joy in that moment. I could drive to church now, I could drive my boys to school and Jayme to his basketball/football practices and games. I was so happy and I felt fine except for the usual side effects from the medications, which was always a concern of mine, especially long term. I was regaining some confidence, despite the anxiety of being shocked twice and the constant fear of it happening again.

My attitude was changing for the better all the time. I was more positive, and people told me how nice it was to be around someone who had been through what I had yet I never complained. I decided to keep trying the dating scene, a coffee/tea here and there. I remember one time when I got dressed up to go out, my youngest son said, "Mom, you don't look like you had a cardiac arrest." Not sure what that would look like, but I guess he was giving me a compliment. It is important to remember that you shouldn't judge a book by its cover. You have no idea what people are going through just by looking at them. I looked completely fine on the outside, but I was struggling at times, day to day with how I felt physically, mentally and emotionally.

While I was on one date with a firefighter, I told him how I'd survived a cardiac arrest and had two shocks from my ICD, he just looked at me seriously and said, "You're hard to kill." I busted out laughing because, thankfully, it was true.

As the weeks flew by, my old saying "I'm still here" when asked how I was doing turned into a very elated "I'm still here!" as I embraced the fact that even though things were not ideal, I was still here to enjoy life as much as possible. This is a perfect example of how sometimes, it is not what you say but how you say it.

I was very blessed to have survived three times now. I had celebrated another birthday, my kids' birthdays, the first day of school and so many other special occasions. I began to really appreciate my device and not be embarrassed about it. It was my lifesaver, and I was finally accepting of it.

My divorce was finalized in the Spring of 2015, and that closure was long overdue. It was important to keep focusing on taking better care of myself, eating right, and exercising, although exercise did scare me because I was afraid to get my heart rate up too high and possibly provoke an arrhythmia. I would typically just walk on my treadmill three to four times a week when I felt I could, without pushing myself too hard. I have low blood pressure which made it difficult to function some days as well, but it was important to keep as active as I could.

I was having a tough time with the weight gain from the steroids, because I was always relatively slim throughout my life, but fortunately I would be taking a break from them which would help with that. It was important that I continued to exercise for my heart, I had to pay attention to my sodium intake, especially with having a heart condition now. I researched adding supplements and vitamins to my routine, but I always had to check to see if anything would interfere with my heart medications. There were so many things I could not take anymore that included some over- the-counter medicines, which can cause heart palpitations. I needed to be wary of these things and to pay attention to everything I put in my body. It's important to understand that everybody's situation is different. There are so many underlying reasons for heart attacks and cardiac arrest. Always follow your doctor's orders and learn as much as you can about your particular situation so you can do what is best for you and your recovery.

The rest of the year went great, I continued to make the most of a not-so-ideal situation and I continued to hope and pray for continued better days ahead.

The following year I got to celebrate my 46th birthday

and so many other important occasions, for which I was so thankful. My health situation had remained stable since 2014 with no shocks or any other issues surrounding my heart condition, which was fantastic. I was able to continue driving and being there for my kids when they needed me. Every day got easier as I started to forget about my condition and focus on all the blessings I had in my life. Mindset is so important and I was determined to make the most of my situation, until I couldn't, that is.

Pure devastation and heartbreak struck our household. Our beloved Chico got sick suddenly and was diagnosed with a form of cancer at the young age of eight years old. Losing him was so painful, it broke our hearts. My kids had been through so much already... a divorce, moving twice, almost losing me three times and now this! We still miss him to this day and I cannot imagine the thought of losing our other dog too. Lexy is going on eleven and she is my heart dog; she doesn't take her eyes off of me. She has some anxiety and I often wonder if it is because of everything I have been through. Lexy is the sweetest girl and hopefully she will be with us for many years to come.

My favourite time of the year was upon us once again; my passion is decorating, and I go all out at Christmastime, but as the end of 2016 was approaching, I was starting to feel another emotion. I was going on year four of being single. I tried to be excited and happy for the holiday season, but it was hard. We were still mourning the loss of Chico and would be for a very long time, but I needed to try to be happy for everyone's sake. As I sat alone for a few hours on Christmas Eve, waiting for my kids to get home, I realized that I did not want to spend another Christmas alone; I had my kids, of course, but I meant without a partner. My boys lived with me full-time and would have visits with their dad throughout the week and on special occasions. It was an arrangement that I cherished because I did not like being away from them for long. They were really all I had.

I made a wish that night that the good Lord would send me my person!

New Year's Eve had come and gone, and I was hopeful for a better 2017! I was ready to let down some walls and be vulnerable. I was over the moon that I had finished off another year with no shocks. Positive thinking and being grateful for all that I had, was always key to looking ahead.

Chapter Five

A NEW BEGINNING

I met John at a restaurant on January 11th, 2017. He had messaged me a couple of times the year before, but I had put him and a few people off because I still had some doubts about the dating scene. It had been disappointment after disappointment, but I refused to give up on the possibility of finding love. I had been meeting very active people and there were days that I could barely walk up the stairs, so it was hard to find my match. I needed someone, active or not, who accepted me and my condition. John was that guy. When I first saw him, I was instantly attracted to him and knew if things went well, I would want to see him again. He is seven years younger than me too… bonus!! Did that mean I was a cougar? We hit it off right away and continued to date on a regular basis.

The first year of our relationship had its challenging moments because, although I was doing well, I was still dealing with some insecurities that were hard to shake. In the beginning of any relationship, you don't really know where it's going. We had a few bumps in the road, but in the end, we worked through all of our issues.

I had thrown a party in late December of that year to celebrate John's 40th birthday, it was nice to have friends and family over because I rarely entertained at home. Unfortunately, I got sick a few weeks after that and John took great care of me. He ended up taking me to emerge after a few days because my throat was so sore, that I couldn't even swallow water. I also had an elevated temperature and was starting to feel very weak. Thankfully I was admitted right away and put on an intravenous drip because I was becoming dehydrated. I was diagnosed with esophageal thrush, I had recently started up on a steroid drug again and wondered if that is what may have caused it. I was released hours later with prescriptions, one being for my throat to numb it, so I would be able to eat and drink. I felt better within days and started to feel like myself again. It was good that we went to the hospital when we did. When you have serious health issues, it is so important to get medical attention right away if you are not feeling well.

John worked away but started to entertain the idea of opening his own business. That would mean he could be home with me every night, instead of being gone for days at a time. I finally had someone I could count on who made me feel like nothing was wrong with me. We became each other's best friend, and we spent all of our time together. I finally realized after all these years, that I deserved happiness, and I was worthy of this kind of love. I thank God all the time for sending me him. So many others did not want to invest their time in me, which was fine; it took the right person to do so.

John and I got engaged in July of 2018, and he moved in with me and my boys. Everything was going great! He had not witnessed anything pertaining to my heart condition, just some weight gain from the steroids that I started taking earlier in the year, because another PET scan indicated active inflammation. The following year John started his own business that he had talked about, and it was so wonderful that he didn't have to travel out of province for work anymore.

We tied the knot on July 11th, 2019 at a local beach. It was just him and me, my boys, and a friend of mine. A justice of the peace married us and it was a beautiful day. I wanted something small and intimate because I had already had the big wedding and did not desire to do that again. John, of course, is so easygoing that he was fine with whatever we did. I was now in the type of marriage everyone longs for; I had met my soulmate and my boys were incredibly happy for us.

A couple of months after we married, my joy turned into complete sadness though when a young man, around my son Jesse's age passed away in a fatal car accident. The accident happened just several feet from where we lived and it woke us up. I was devastated and my heart hurt terribly for the family. I often drove by where the accident happened and realized after it did, how if there had been guardrails on both sides of the road, things may have turned out differently. I was bothered by this so much that I reached out to my local municipal councillor, and through several emails to her, she made it happen! The guardrails were installed within a couple of months. I was so happy and thankful to her for that, but wished that they had already been there. I've always been an empath, very sensitive and compassionate but I've noticed that since I almost died, I'm even more so. Having a near death experience makes you realize so much more just how precious life really is. My thoughts have remained with that family indefinitely.

In the beginning of 2020, we had to move because the homeowner wanted to sell the property we were renting. I was so happy we had John in our lives now because moving again was not something we were looking forward to, especially when it wasn't our idea. He and my boys moved all of our belongings, which made things so much easier for me. I don't know what I would do without my three J's, they are my everything! The rental we moved into wasn't ideal, but it was all we could find at the time. It was unusual that the landlord made us sign a five-month fixed lease. I had never heard of something like that before; it is usually yearly or month to month. We did not care for the place but figured we would be there for a year and then try to buy a house. Then COVID hit. Oh my, what a time that was, being stuck in our homes, life -changing for sure. We followed all protocols… handwashing, sanitizer, mask wearing, and thankfully got through it unscathed.

We had celebrated my 50th birthday at home, just me, John, my boys and my girl, Lexy. It was not the 50th birthday celebration most people hope for, but I was alive and beyond thankful to spend it with the loves of my life, it couldn't get much better that that, it was perfect!

One day in June, while doing outside work for a client, my husband overheard her talking to someone on the phone about her rental coming available on August 1st. John questioned her about it because our lease was up at the end of July. Long story short, we rented his client's home. It was like it was meant to be because it was available the same time our lease ended. The new place was closer to my youngest son's school. It was ten times nicer, newer, less rent, and it had more bathrooms and a garage… jackpot! We were extremely excited to move this time, but our goal of home ownership was always on our minds… until the unbelievable real estate market took effect, that is. I am sure many dreams were shattered then. It seemed like everyone wanted to move to Nova Scotia and were willing to pay an arm and a leg for real estate. We had no choice but to put home ownership on the back burner, and we settled in nicely in our beautiful rental. Life was good, the kids were happy and healthy, and John's business was doing well.

I took some time to focus on some at-home courses I was taking, which involved home decorating/design and staging. I had become certified in interior decorating/design and was looking to expand on that. The knowledge learned from my courses could help John with his business or allow me to start something on my own someday. I had a lot of time on my hands still, so I tried to keep my mind busy.

It had been six long wonderful years since I'd had my last shock, and I was feeling more comfortable and more at ease all the time. I may have been too comfortable at times with not watching what I ate, or my activity level. These things were not always at the top of my priority list as much as they should have been.

My EF had gone up a little bit over the years which made me happy, but one of my cardiologists felt it would never be close to normal again because of the extent of scarring on my heart. There is no cure for cardiac sarcoidosis, it is a condition that can be active or inactive at times, but it is one that I have to live with and have it treated accordingly. I still suffered side effects of course from the meds and the inability to do all the things I wanted to do, but life was good considering all things…

Chapter Six

HERE WE GO AGAIN

It was 2021; and the world as we knew it had changed. We were still living in the COVID-19 pandemic. Businesses were closing; friends and family relationships were breaking up because of the divide in beliefs and choices. It was really a sad situation. Many lives were lost, and people were forever changed. Fortunately we were not affected by the pandemic too much, other than being restricted like everyone else with what we could or could not do at varying times. Not being able to spend time with family on special occasions was hard, and my husband, who is from Newfoundland, had not seen his family since 2019. We didn't lose anyone to COVID-19, and we were incredibly thankful about that of course. My heart went out to all those affected negatively by these unprecedented times.

We continued to live our lives as best as we could. My boys and husband worked when they were able to, and we continued to think positively and hope for the best. Jesse started university and moved out that year. This was a difficult time for me; but I was happy for him, he was not living far from me so that made me feel better.

My boys were getting older, twenty-one and sixteen years old to be exact… *Where did the time go?* I was always so grateful that I could stay home with them, and my health issues allowed me to continue doing so. I had often been accused, by some, of caring and doing too much, of being too strict, and I had been told to cut the umbilical cord many times. That is hard to do when your life revolves around your kids. Even harder, when you were almost taken from them, you cherish every little thing even more. I had always put them first, and the only thing I was guilty of was loving them too much. As long as I am on this Earth, I can never do too much for my boys, but I do understand how important it is to put yourself first too. John was the one who taught me to not care what others think or say. I had always worn my heart on my sleeve and things bothered me easily. He is my rock in everything; he has my back, and I have his.

Things continued to go well, considering what we were living through. John and I celebrated our 2nd wedding anniversary on July 11th and we would visit the spot where we got married on occasion. We both liked the simple things in life and just a quiet dinner and some alone time was all that was needed.

On Friday, July 20th; just nine days after our

anniversary, my husband and I were watching a movie like we did most weekend evenings. My son Jayme was at work until 11p.m., and I went to pick him up when he was off. John would usually go but I wanted to on this particular night. I brought Jayme home and continued to watch the movie with John. Just after it turned midnight, as I was sitting on the couch next to him, I started to get dizzy, and my vision was blacking out. I yelled out his name and then I was gone. I jolted awake seconds later and felt a hot sensation around my device; I was scared and understandably very shook up. My third shock now, and my poor husband did not know what to do. He told me that when I was out, he was slapping my face, trying to get me to come to. I told him in the future that shouldn't be necessary. After he consoled me and calmed me down, he drove me to the hospital. I knew from previous experiences that when you have a shock you should go to the hospital as soon as you can. I was seen immediately and admitted to the cardiac floor by early morning. I knew what this meant… no driving for six months! Although I was devastated about that; I was so thankful that this episode had not happened an hour earlier behind the wheel, while I was picking up my son.

All my shocks have been appropriate shocks, meaning they were administered because they were needed. Had they not worked, I would not be alive to write this book and would have missed out on so many special occasions over the years. I have encountered episodes where I was just two beats away from a shock and didn't realize it because my ICD paced me out of it. This has happened in my sleep, and I did not know it until I had my ICD interrogated and the technician told me. It was scary for me to find that out. From time to time, I feel palpitations which are scary as well. It is an ongoing thing to deal with, but things could always be worse is what I tell myself. Because I have passed out in the past before I receive a shock, I know that if I have a dizzy spell in the future, I should try to sit if I am standing, as to prevent a fall.

I had experienced a very quick blackout while I was driving a couple of months prior to this latest shock, but it was only for a split second and then I was fine. This was terrifying, because if my ICD had not corrected the arrhythmia, it could have led to an accident and a shock. I was shaken up after that incident but because it happened so quickly, I was able to continue driving home, and thankfully I didn't have far to go. It took me several days before I could drive because I was afraid that it might happen again. I had to muster up the courage and tell myself that I couldn't worry about something that might not happen, it was like getting knocked off a horse and getting right back on. Not wanting to endanger other's lives is what I was most concerned about. I should've realized something was off at that time, but it wasn't discovered what that was, until after I had my shock on the 20th.

There was talk about putting me on the antiarrhythmic drug but only if it happened again, they decided. I was happy to hear that because my intent is to not to take it anymore. After getting my blood work done, they discovered my dosage for my thyroid was too high and they felt that could have been the reason I had the arrhythmia. Right away, they changed the dosage and informed me to get my thyroid checked every three months going forward.

The last few years I had been going for checkups every six months and things had been stable during that time. I had to have the occasional PET scan done over the years to see if there was any active inflammation, but this wasn't required at this time because of the thyroid issue. I have been on a continual low maintenance dose of steroids over the last few years to keep inflammation at bay, in hopes to avoid any arrhythmias. My thyroid and eyesight had started being affected when I was on the antiarrhythmic drug before. As I mentioned, the drug has some side effects, so I was incredibly happy it was not recommended at that time. I am thankful for the meds I take as they keep me going but I am not happy about the side effects, I have not investigated any other methods and I am not against that; I just have always taken my medications that are prescribed to me. I take them when they are supposed to be taken, and I listen to my cardiologist's recommendations.

Every time I have a shock from my ICD, it sets me

back. It takes me to that depressive state where I feel sorry for myself, and I wish yet again that this never happened to me. It is certainly not the life I envisioned or wanted but it is what I am dealing with, and I cannot change it. It is no different than anyone else who is dealing with a life-threatening disease or any kind of health issue. We are usually at the mercy of our illness. Figuring out how to live with it is the most important thing we can do, along with never giving up. Your health is paramount to anything else. Without it, what can you do? It does not matter how much money you may have, because if you cannot do anything, then what is the point of it all? This condition was not a result of something I did. It happened to me for whatever reason, just like many other diseases that people have. I will probably never know how or why exactly, but at this point it doesn't matter; I can't change it.

It is so important that I keep my diet and exercise regimen in check, so I started to incorporate dance and low impact aerobics into my weekly routine, when I could. I have some chronic pain in my legs and hips which makes it difficult to be consistent with exercising. I've always had a love of music and dance, so listening to my favorite songs made exercising more enjoyable on the good days, and I looked forward to it. Exercise and eating a proper diet are the best things you can do for your body, especially if you have heart disease.

Jesse and Jayme were always champions throughout

everything, they are strong and never let what was happening to me affect their own lives and mindsets. I am so proud of my boys, they are hard workers, they do good in school and they never cause me any problems. I had been concerned about them over the years, but they are doing great and I am so blessed to have them.

I am a SURVIVOR! I got up one more time, dusted myself off and was thankful yet again that I had another chance at life, even if I could not drive until January of 2022. This scenario was all too familiar…

Chapter Seven

FAITH OVER FEAR

I have been through more ordeals than I would like to admit. I've survived hardships, divorce, the extremely difficult effects of heart disease and many hurts and losses. I have lost touch with many people over the years, because I became a bit of a recluse. I spent a lot of time by myself, and I got used to it. I truly am a homebody and love surrounding myself with beautiful things decorwise. I love before and afters and cannot wait until we own a house someday so I can utilize my creative talents to make it our perfect forever home.

Living with heart disease has been very scary at times; wondering when I might have another shock is even scarier, but it is something I cannot control. I always remind myself of the serenity prayer and say it often…

'God, grant me the serenity to accept the things I cannot change, courage to change the things I can, and wisdom to know the difference.'

I live my life one moment at a time and one day at a time. I know that life is precious, and it can be taken away from you anytime, anywhere. I surround myself with beautiful things, I try to be as positive as I can, and I frown on negativity or anyone trying to upset my apple cart. I cannot deal with toxicity like I used to. I do not want to. Our days are numbered, and I want the time I have left to be as enjoyable as possible. I know it is not realistic to think everything is always going to be okay all the time, but it works for me, and I will continue to tell myself that it will be. After having four chances at life, I often wonder if that cat bite has given me nine lives… if so, I guess I must have five left now. Whatever I have left, it will be spent with my loved ones, praying daily and thanking God for all he does for me in this life.

I live in faith over fear, I choose to be happy, I choose to accept what is and change what I can. I do not know what the future holds, and yes, that is scary too, but whatever it is, I will manage it to the best of my ability. I do get down at times when it comes to past mistakes, I am only human, but I must remind myself that the key word here is past. I cannot change anything that was; I can only look forward, take each day as it comes, be thankful for it and pray and hope for a better tomorrow.

People in my situation know what it is like to live in fear of that next shock, hoping it doesn't happen again, and wondering when it might. This can take a lot out of you and steal so much of your joy in the present tense.

Some people feel the shock first which I am sure can be very painful. I, however, have gone unconscious first, so I have not felt any shocks from my ICD. I have, however, heard a solid, few seconds long tone coming from my device before, which concerned me, but it turned out that I had a magnet too close to it. Magnets will deactivate an ICD, so it is important to be mindful of that. You will hear a beeping tone after you have a shock and you will hear that as well if the battery is getting low, in which case you should have your battery tested.

Living in anxiety and depression is one of the most difficult things to endure. Because of my faith, I have been able to control the extent of those things. Not everyone feels the same, and my heart goes out to those who find it difficult to live in that mindset. I will say that time helps, time heals and with time you do worry less. Having a support system is so important too, to help you through those tough times. I struggle with weight gain at times still, the meds and lack of energy makes this easy, but I try to continue to be mindful of what I am eating and to move more. It is a continuous battle.

My wish for anyone going through difficult times, no matter what they are, is that you truly take the time to be thankful for any of the good you still have in your life. I have felt down and out many times, but I did not stay there. I can still do so many things, so you must look at what you can still do too. There is a saying: "Every day above ground is a great day." That is so true. You still have time: time to be with the ones you love; time to see them; time to talk to them, hold them, love them, whatever the case may be. Do I wish this never happened to me? Of course, one thousand times over, but it did, and I will be okay. I have been given years with my children that I might not have had otherwise, for that alone, I am beyond blessed. It has changed me but not for the worse. It has taught me how strong I can be and how fragile and important life is, and to have a grateful heart.

I rarely think about my condition anymore. At times I get sad, yes, because I do not know what the future holds – none of us do – but it does not consume me like it used to. I do not focus on my ICD either; I have accepted both. I am not looking forward to the day that I will have to have my device replaced, but I have three and a half years of battery life left. ICDs are operated by a battery and the device needs to be replaced when it is getting low; this can happen anytime up to ten years or longer. I will deal with that when the time comes and be fine. I can drive again, so that is exciting!. It has been over a year since my last shock! I try not to think about it happening again and how I would lose my right to drive. I look at the positives, I am not on a transplant list for a new heart, because my condition has remained stable over the years, despite the number of shocks I have had. This is great news that I hope will continue for many years to come.

My heart is damaged, but it still works. It can love

and be loved, and I found my true love. Forgive yourself for anything you need to and forgive others; it frees you from pain and frustration. Life is beautiful. Life is too short. Live it, love it; it is a true gift. Be thankful and grateful for all you have. Tell those you love how you feel; show them too. Most of us only get one chance at this thing called life. I thank God every day for what I have and pray for what I need or want. He is my light when it is dark. Always focus on the good, not the bad; the difference between a good day and a bad day is your attitude. You've got this…

My wish for anyone reading this book is that somehow, you find comfort in my story and my survival. Never give up because there is always hope. Think positive, accept what is and change what you can, and try not to worry about something that may never happen. That is wasted energy.

I am forever grateful for the care I have received from my cardiologists and nurses who took great care of me during my hospital stays and who continue to take great care of me; they are on this journey with me and others alike. They are the true heroes in this world; and so is my Jesse. Saving lives is a superpower!

Chapter Eight

THE GIFT OF WAKING UP

Do you ever just stop and think for a moment how precious your life is? Do you spend your days being thankful that you're alive, or do you take it for granted? Do you find beauty and appreciation in the simple things, or is your life consumed with obtaining more of the things that don't matter? Do you realize that if you woke up today… you are blessed!

> This is the day the Lord has made; let us rejoice
> and be glad in it -Psalm 118:24

Chapter seven was supposed to be the last chapter of this book before I was to publish it, but having a fourth shock changed that. On October 14th, 2022; I awoke at 7 a.m. like I do most mornings. I saw my son off to school and then went back to bed because I was still tired; a good night's sleep is a luxury that I'm not accustomed to unfortunately. At approximately 8:40 a.m. I sat up suddenly from my slumber and felt like something was wrong. I immediately called out to my husband to come here, and I explained to him how I felt and what my concern was. I thought that maybe my ICD either paced me out of an arrhythmia or I received a shock from it; I prayed that the latter wasn't the case. I called the device clinic to ask them to do a remote transmission so they could tell me what happened, if anything! I had to leave a message because nobody answered, so I waited patiently to hear back from someone. Approximately a half an hour later, my phone rang.

The lady on the other end said, "Did you know you had a shock this morning?"

My heart sank. All I remember was her asking me if I could come to the hospital. I hung up the phone and cried like a baby in my husband's arms. I can tell you that no matter how many times this happens, my initial reaction, is utter devastation. I was so upset that I couldn't drive for six months, assuming…that is, that nothing else happens again, before then. The one thing that I couldn't stop thinking about was, *what if my ICD didn't work?* Those thoughts were upsetting me even more, and for a little while I was afraid to go to sleep. I can tell you wholeheartedly that this device in my chest is EVERYTHING! I am here because of it, I got to see another day. There is no luck at all in my survival, luck is about things happening by chance. I am still here for a reason and so are you. Whether you have an ICD or not, if you wake up in the morning, that is one of the greatest gifts you could ever receive.

For several days, I remained upset and nervous. It is okay to feel the devastation but moving on from it is key to living a happy and fulfilling life. I picked myself up again, calmed my inner negative, worrying thoughts and reminded myself that this wasn't my first rodeo, and this too shall pass. I had to have the usual tests done, of course, and a PET scan was ordered to see if there was any active inflammation in and around my heart. It turned out that there was only inflammation in my esophagus, which wasn't surprising because I had been dealing with a lot of acid reflux over the last year. A second scope of my esophagus was ordered because the last one had been well over a year ago. My thoughts began to sway from my heart to my esophagus, I had learned that one of the drugs I was on could cause some issues with it. Just something else I could worry about, or I could take my own advice and pray on it, be still, and think positively. There was some discussion about changing one of my heart medications too which I wasn't thrilled about because as I mentioned earlier, I don't like trying new- to- me medications. Side effects are always a concern, especially ones that may cause severe adverse reactions. I feel strongly that people should educate themselves on what they are taking, make changes in their lifestyles to help with their health issues, and to keep an open conversation going with their health care providers about treatment.

When I look in the mirror, I see a brave and extremely strong person. I have endured more than I could've ever imagined, and I hope whoever is reading this book sees the same thing, when they look in the mirror as well. Struggles and challenges strengthen you. You cannot grow without them, pain is so hard in the moment but with time, it eases. We are always stronger than we think we are. Out of your growth, determination and persistence in overcoming all your trials and tribulations…you inspire others. You become more compassionate because you know what it's like to be at your lowest. Write out that bucket list and design that vision board, you are still here for a reason. Love the life you have and the skin you live in, things may not be perfect, or how you hoped they would be, but they could always be worse!

I continue to have an attitude of gratitude always, even on the not-so-great days. On those days, I just remind myself how I'm still here to enjoy this gift of life I was given. I must dig deep some days and know that my survival story is not over, I will continue fighting until my time is up. I had been reminded once again that I can have a shock at anytime…it could be within days, weeks, months, years or never? (That is wishful thinking) I honestly try very hard not to think about it, having palpitations makes this difficult at times, but keeping my mind occupied on other things is vital to moving forward from the setbacks. I am grateful in each waking moment, and I appreciate the gift of waking up more than anything.

I am looking forward to my favorite time of year again, how blessed I am to celebrate another Christmas! This is where my focus lies these days, and where it should. As long as I'm here, I will enjoy each day as best as I can and thank God for his blessings, especially the 'waking up' one!

My health journey will continue and I will remain grateful in it. I have been so blessed to still be here with my loved ones close to me. That's what life is all about, spending time with the ones you love. Next year, I WILL drive again!

God bless,

With love, hope and many prayers,

Your heart friend